FUNDAMENTALS OF NUTRITION
In The Light Of Spiritual Science

FUNDAMENTALS OF NUTRITION
In The Light Of Spiritual Science

By

G. F. MIER AND H. HOOGEWERFF

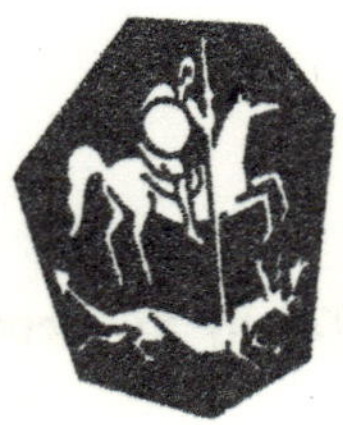

St. George Publications

Spring Valley, New York

TABLE OF CONTENTS

I. PREFATORY NOTE

The articles and essays included in this book were first published in the last year or two of World War II and in the few years immediately following. In spite of the dire situation prevailing at that time in Holland, Mrs. Hoogewerff's native land, and in Great Britain, Mrs. Mier's home, a certain note of hope and optimism penetrate them. This although there were constant shortages of food, fuel, shelter and clothing.

Because we wished to tamper as little as possible with what both authors wrote, an occasional word or turn of phrase may seem strange or unusual. Occasionally, we have changed the name of a vegetable from its English or Continental name as it appeared in the original article to its more familiar (here in the United States) American name.

It is the publisher's hope that, through the information presented here, a Nutrition cognizant of Man as a Being of Body, Soul and Spirit will more and more come into being throughout the English-speaking world.

II. FUNDAMENTALS OF COOKING

by Gertrude Mier

1. THE THREEFOLD NATURE OF PLANT AND MAN

When as gardeners or farmers we search for ideas about cooking, as new and living as those we apply on the land—lest what is well begun in field and garden be wasted and undone in our kitchens—we can do no better than follow the poet Schiller's advice:

"Seekest Thou the Highest, the Greatest, Behold the Plant it can teach Thee!"

Let us then go out into nature and look at the plant with open eyes and hearts, for all our kitchen work has to take its start out there.

One of the most fundamental principles of cooking can be learned from the very form of the plant organism, if we let this form itself speak to us. What is the chief characteristic of a plant, of a garden flower, a cabbage or a turnip? The green leaf—tentatively at first unfolding its small simple lobes and spreading out into more and more complex and varied forms when the stem rises higher above the ground on its way towards the light. Suddenly the plant then draws its form together again and with the forming of the flowerbud enters upon an entirely new stage of development: the flower. This shows quite new qualities: manifold colors, scent, aroma. Here, in stamen and pistil, the plant turns more inward, becomes more involved, when it prepares the goal and end of its life in seed- and fruit-formation.

Flower and leaf reveal their forms openly to our eyes in sun and air above the ground, but we are also aware of the fact that within the soil is the third organ, the root. In time this is actually the first organ of the plant, and it grows downward, towards the center of the earth, away from the surface of the soil, before the first leaves, the cotelydons, are sent up towards the sun. The element of the root is the cool, moist, dark earth, just as the flower lives in the elements of warmth and light above, and the green leaves unfold their activity in the realm between. Their weaving interplay and interchange hold together in unity that which is torn asunder in the polarities of above and below, of wet and dry, of condensed and dispersed, hard and soft, cold and warm, darkness and light, earth and heavens.

A threefold being is the plant with root, leaf and flower, and the whole meaning of the plant's seasonal life is to bring into living harmony what the ground below and the heavens above can bestow. Out of the duality of root and flower, the leaf creates the life of the threefold plant organism.

Thus it is also with man who, like the plant, has a threefold body. With his feet he stands on the earth and moves over it; his head is carried above, freely to look around and to face the world; and the middle part of his body, the chest, keeps the two poles in harmony.

The differences are naturally great, for man is a far more complex being, endowed with soul and spirit. His threefoldness is therefore also more elaborate and involved, because his body has to be the home of an individual spirit and has to be the expression of thinking, feeling and willing. But wherever we study his body, in the structure of skeleton and muscles, or in the organs and their functions, this threefoldness appears again and again. We can observe it in the closed, round form of the head, simple in outline, hard and mineralized: or in the open, manifold shapes of pelvis and limbs and in the rib formation between, forming a closed chest towards the head, but opening up into the more mobile lower ribs. We can see it in the forming of the muscles, which cover the head tightly with little inclination towards soft flesh, while in the lower organism stronger and more fleshy muscles appear. We also find it in the inner organs. The head is the center of our nerve-sense-system with the brain's beautiful structure and the five main senses. Here we are fully awake, here we like to be cool and keep our head quiet and still, for here observing and thinking find their earthly, bodily instruments. The lower organism harbors the main organs of the metabolic processes of digestion and reproduction, of movement—the organs on which our will depends. This part of the body needs warmth for its well being.

In between, in the middle of our body, are lungs and heart, where all interchange takes place between the air without and within through our breathing, and between the metabolism and warmth of below and above, where in rhythm of blood and breathing head and limbs are in living contact. The essence of our being, the ego, weaves and lives on the stream of the blood and through our feeling connects thinking and willing harmoniously.

Threefold man has head, heart and limbs which correspond to the root, leaf and flower of the threefold plant. The similarity and correspondence of this threefoldness can be seen in many more and wonderful details: Man has hairs, the plant has "hair" roots. The plant's leaves are "heart" shaped. Man's lungs when opened up look like real trees with trunk, branches, and leaves—to mention only a few examples.

Man is the plant "upside down," or the plant is man "downside up." Were the sun within the earth, the plant would have the same direction as man, and the flowers would be underground; were man still dependent on the outer sun, he would have to stand on his head.

What is the lesson the cook can learn from such a picture of plant and man? That threefold man needs to have represented in his food all three parts of the plant. We need the roots* so that our head may be built up in such a way that thinking finds a useful tool in the brain. We need the flower and fruit for all metabolic processes to function well. The leaf strengthens and supports the rhythmic processes in us without which the body would be unbalanced. Examples of menus and recipes are given which take this rule into account and show how the threefold plant can be represented on the menus of our chief meal of the day. Another chapter will bring further ways and means of creating the threefold plant itself during the cooking process. There are many possibilities of establishing the harmonious interplay of the light-warmth–(flower–) pole of the plant and the dark-cold–(root–) pole. But however we achieve this, the satisfaction, the health, the nourishment we derive from our meals will be endlessly greater when we take the plant's lesson very seriously and follow this golden, fundamental rule of cooking in all we do with our food. There is no exception from this rule, with or without meat, its observance creates a better meal and often makes the dullest stomach-filler into real food, fit for the threefold organism of man. Man's head, chest and limbs need the plant's root, leaf and flower so that man may find through the food in his body an adequate home on earth for his truly human activity.

This threefold harmony on earth as revealed by the plant is but a small earthly reflection of a divine revelation as it streams down to earth on Christmas Eve in the greeting of the Angel. Here we find it again in its heavenly origin: "Glory to God in the Highest, Peace on Earth to Men of Good Will." Between the glory of the starry heavens above and men of good will on earth lies the Christ child in heart's cradle, bringing peace to earth and living harmony between all that lives above and all that is below. Our cooking, our routine work in the kitchen will be redeemed and inspired, if a ray of this Christmas Greeting is allowed to shine into our kitchens; then it will bring a still greater meaning to the golden cooking rule which we have learned from the plant.

"Seekest Thou the Highest, the Greatest, Behold, the Plant it can teach Thee!"

---

*This holds good only for true roots; tubers like potatoes or Jerusalem artichokes are swollen parts of stem, sunk below the ground and have different qualities.

2. THE SEVEN TASTES

In our search for further instructions about cooking, we can again go to the plant and ask it to teach us another lesson. Watching its growth from the seed in the ground to the blossom unfolding in sun and air, we find that the cool, dark ground gives to the subterranean part of the plant, the root, and all that lives in this sphere the tendency to be firm and mineralized. This pole contracts everything, it hardens substances and forms, gives heaviness and weight.

The plant, however, does not fall entirely under the spell of the gravity forces. It frees itself from the pull of the earth, grows upwards towards the surrounding sphere. Here, in sunlight and air the influences are quite contrary. An uplifting and dispersing process takes place, hard substance is dissolved, form is loosened and expanded. What is held fast and firm below, is opened up and freed above. We see this in root and blossom, in the way in which the leaves change from the plain, simple, unserrated cotelydon lobes to the finely cut leaves higher up on the stem. Even the color goes through the same metamorphosis from the dull white or grey of the root, to the green of the leaf and lastly to the many colored petals of the flower.

This life of the plant between the pole of darkness and the pole of light, this struggle between the polarities of the gravity-bound root and the light-freed blossom, finds still another expression in taste and flavor, in scent and aroma which the plant develops in varied forms in different parts of its body. This is a finer, more intimate conversation, so to speak, between the plant and the cosmic and terrestrial forces, than that which we can directly see with our eyes or touch with our hands in form and substance. And yet: the tastes show the same polarities out of which the plant weaves its life.

In order to understand these elusive qualities called taste more deeply we may try to order them, but find it hard to get hold of them in concept and experience, for tastes are only partly manifested in physical material form. The names "ethereal," "volatile," oils, which are bearers of tastes, hint at this fact. Perhaps we do best to follow the old classification of Aristotle's which comprises all shades and nuances in the following tastes: bitter, harsh, acid, salty, sharp, oily and sweet. These seven main tastes appear in the plant in different parts and we shall try to assign them to their natural places. Some of them are more akin to warmth and light, to all that wants to expand and dissolve into the surrounding sphere. The uppermost realm of the plant, blossom and fruit, are their rightful home. There is first and foremost the sweet flavor which the plant usually develops in the warmth of the sun, in its heavenly pole. Fruit and nuts have natural sweetness, and the bees produce sweet honey out of the nectar of the blossom. Next we have to put the oily taste, which is not usually classified among flavors, but little though we may be conscious of it, deeper consideration will show that it is a quality of its own, and not only the bearer of subtle flavors. This also develops under the expanding influence of the warmth pole, and much oil is found in seeds and nuts, in the fruits or in the wax of their skin.

These two are entirely free of all earthbound, hardening influences, but the sharp, hot taste, in spite of the fire which shows it as a child of the sun, stands already more under the force of gravity. Expansion and dispersion are no longer alone at work, we find traces of the earth's pull in the biting of the sharpness. Peppers and mustards, the chief sources of hot flavors live, however, right at the top of the plant.

How very different are the earthbound tastes, those which stand entirely under the influence of the hardening, contracting forces of gravity and earth: bitter and harsh. They belong to the pole of darkness in the plant, the root, as we can see in dandelion, chickory, gentian and others. These tastes contract our mouth and pull us together when we taste them. Harsh is already a little milder and reaches up towards the stem of the plant, while bitter belongs to the very bottom, the root. Acid (or sour) too has strongly contracting properties, as well we know, but we find it in the plant already in the leaves.

There remains only one taste, the salty, which from our point of view, has to be placed in the center. Salt is meant here entirely as taste, as we become conscious of it in our mouth; salt in this sense does not stand for the mineral, crystal, or substance, but only for that taste which is neither dissolving, nor contracting. Belonging to the very center of the plant, to the region of leaf and stalk it balances the polarities. Nay, it even puts them into their right places, through its mere presence, and calls forth their very own nature in the other flavors. Therefore it is the most essential of all tastes, as indispensible in sweet as in savory dishes. There comes to our mind the Bible word: When now the salt has lost its flavor wherewith shall it be salted? And Mark (Chap. IX, v. 50) continues the word: Have salt within you and peace one with another. Besides all the deep, sublime meanings of this mystery word, it also throws light on such a simple cooking lesson. The salt in our dishes brings peace, harmony, balance into all tastes, from bitter to sweet; it orders them and strengthens their own qualities.

Quite naturally then these seven tastes fall again into a threefold unity: Sweet, oily and sharp belong to the light—or flower pole of the plant, to the heavenly, expanding sphere; bitter, harsh and acid to the darkness—the root pole, the earthly, contracting sphere; and the salt, as balancer and mediator, stands in the middle, like the leaf harmonising both contrasting polarities.

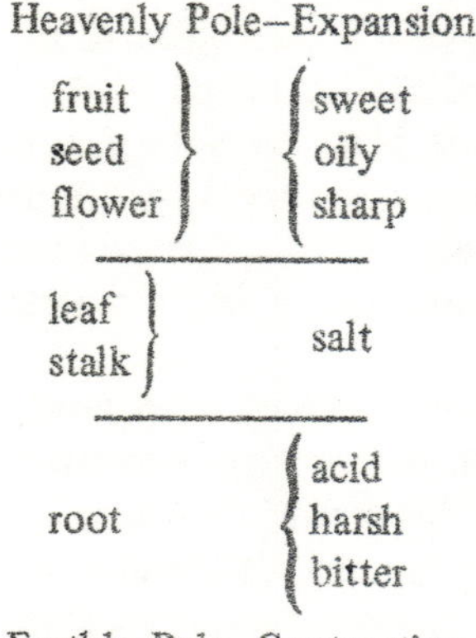

When we order the tastes thus according to the three different plant regions, we may find contradictions in nature, for life does not allow itself to be classified so simply. Many plants have sweet roots, and much bitterness can be found in fruits and nuts. Then we must remember that most plants, and specially those we eat, are onesided in their nature, have often been made so by man for his own ends, and benefit. The carrot or beet have drawn the heavenly sphere right down to their roots, and therefore besides sweetness also bright color appears. Bitterness has shot up into the top of the plant in peppers, in almonds, and acidity appears in fruits and berries. Most of these food plants have sacrificed and neglected some realms, concentrating so to speak (often also in size), on one particular organ or region. We shall find in such cases that this one organ then also becomes the gathering point of all seven tastes. Many of the herbs, e.g., accumulate all tastes in their tiny leaves; yes, they have become so much bearer of taste only, that size, color, beauty are pushed into the background. Spices, herbs, and also vegetable plants, rarely show one simple taste; many of these are mingled and mixed even in a cabbage leaf. It needs great consciousness and practice to learn to differentiate subtle shades and fine nuances of tastes. We have become too apt to look for quantity also in taste, and too lazy and inert to pay attention to their infinite variability and manifoldness.

A good cook will find that she can season dishes well only when she has taught herself the art of tasting the seven flavors separately even there where they appear highly mixed, as in a fennel leaf or caraway seed. A meal is fully satisfactory only inasmuch as our whole threefold body feels equally addressed by the seven tastes in their entirety. We have then again the threefold plant represented in our food, not in substance this time, as was the case with root, leaf, fruit, but in mere quality, as flavor, as taste.

These seven tastes in their influence upon man bring to him all the qualities from the spheres which are their natural home. Sweet and oily have expanding effect upon man, they make him round and placid. The small child, which is still resting in the heavenly sphere and should not be harshly brought down to earth, has a preference for them. Bitter, biting, harsh and sour tend to contract, make hard and lean, even shock us into awakeness, to the awareness of our existence on earth. Old people with their senses already numbed like them, the phlegmatic temperament needs them, while the melancholic who always has his eyes too much down towards the earth can be helped by the tastes of the heavenly sphere, sweet and oily.

But on the whole, we must say, that man on earth needs all seven; all are of equal importance to him, for we must neither lose ourselves in the beauty of the heavens, nor must we become hardened and earthbound through the pull of the earth's gravity. And for our well being it is more important than we realize, that the tastes are carefully balanced in our menus and in our dishes. Naturally they need not be present in equal strength and quantity. One dish, like a pudding or cake is predominately sweet, but even the sweetest dish will nourish better if salt and earthbound tastes are also present, follow the sweet so to speak at least at a distance. Salads and curries, vegetable stews may be savory food, but sweetness should not be entirely absent. The composition of a good menu can become a true picture of how man should place himself into the world. The soup, a salty, savory course, will stimulate us, awaken our interest. The middle course then opens up the whole variety of life and nature; it can bring great manifoldness of tastes, even if the savory will be dominating. Yet, some sweetness in direct form, as chutney, currant jelly, apple sauce, dried fruit is often present, definitely more so than in the soup course. In the dessert, however, the sweet taste rules supreme, filling us with contentment and satisfaction, yes even with the wish for relaxation. The bitterness of the coffee, can then counteract this sleepiness which would make us too unwilling and lazy for work; yet we may sweeten it again in order to make the transition easier to the demands of the life on earth. Thus in the whole menu as well as in the single course or dish the symphony of tastes should be well played through the art in which we bring about their presence and distribution. And whether we give the heavenly pole of sweetness, or the earthly pole of bitterness, preponderance we must never forget, that all six sisters should accompany the one taste, and that none should be left in isolation. Then we have again created a second threefold plant which accompanies root, leaf and fruit, and threefold man will feel still more fully and truly satisfied.

These practical cooking considerations of harmonizing our dishes, of overcoming onesidedness and of balancing polarities, may be rightly put in front of the majestic picture of the great Easter drama, shown to us by Rudolf Steiner in his Statue of the Representative of Mankind. Here the Christ stands in the center, his out-stretched left arm keeping Lucifer in his place and his right hand showing Ahriman the Earth as his rightful realm. A picture of perfect balance and harmony, showing man his great task on earth: to find the way to peace between the Luciferic powers which want to tear him away from the earth into the beauty of heavenly clouds and the Ahrimanic powers which want to harden and fetter him to the Earth. Man is only Man when he succumbs to neither, when he stands firm between the two great polarities and does not allow them to enter the Middle realm. We can then indeed become "the Salt of the Earth."

In the previous considerations about cooking we have drawn knowledge from the picture of the plant as it develops form and qualities during its life and growth between the great polarities of heaven and earth. After we have now chosen from among the plants in our kitchen garden what we need as fruit, leaf and root, when we have carefully planned the flavoring, we must further ask ourselves how rightly to cook them. We have got from the plant some guiding lines about the right type of foodstuffs, let us now seek farther afield in Nature in order to gain advice about the right ways and methods of cooking.

Ancient wisdom, seen in the light of Anthroposophy, can help us here. The Greeks differentiated between four elements underlying all created matter as primeval essence or principle: Fire-Air-Water-Earth. Wherever we deal with matter, with substance, these four are present and active in various ways and combinations; they determine the outer appearance and manifestation of substance. The word "element" is not used in the way of modern chemistry, where it designates the smallest material particle. These elements are also not identical with the forms of aggregate, which are merely their accompanying external effect. "Fire" in this sense is not the flame we see, but all phenomena of warmth and heat. "Air" is not only the air of the atmosphere, but anything that is airy and gaseous. "Water" stands for all liquid and fluid and "Earth" for what is hard, solid, heavy and formed.

We can readily recognize again how matter manifests differently according to the realm of forces in which it develops and we see how two of these elements, Fire and Air, belong to the heavenly pole of expansion, of lightness or levity, of dynamic movement towards the circumference. They tend to flee the earth, to break and dissolve fixed form, to free from bonds anything that comes under their influence.

Water, still vague in form and of flowing movement, obeys already the forces of gravity and falls down upon the ground. It has more solidity and yields to the form of its surroundings. Earth is the prototype of the Earthly pole of contraction; it is all solidity, gravity and rigid, fixed form. From the Fire to the element Earth we see a gradual coming about of form, an arresting of movement into hard solidity, and all matter is thus an expression of an interplay of these elements. The more Fire and Air have worked upon it, the finer and lighter and more mobile it becomes. The more Water and Earth have exerted their influence, the firmer and heavier it will be.

Which part then do these four elements play in the kitchen? What can we learn from their study about the different methods and processes of cooking? At first thought Fire seems to be of paramount importance; for the cooker, the range is the very center of activity in our kitchen. The Sun itself is fire and with its help calls the plants into existence. When we now take the plant out of its natural life cycle into our kitchens, it is understandable that we call upon the fire as our first helper, for cooking is nothing but a continuation of the Sun's work. The plant in nature is freed from the dark, hard soil by the Sun, is pulled up by it into the heavenly sphere, there to mature and ripen. This work of ripening and fruiting is finished in the kitchen through the fire process on our range. As the sun has lifted up the substance of the earth in the plants to a higher, a lighter stage, more akin to our own bodily substances, so we continue this process to still further stages. Through cooking, matter is raised higher that it may not be felt as an alien intruder, a slight poison, that it may easily be assimilated by the human being in his digestive processes.

The thought that we imitate and continue the Sun's way of working is a helpful directive and tells us how much and what kind of cooking should be done, whether roasting, stewing, boiling or frying is indicated. The Sun, when allowed to work longer upon the plant, after fruit and seed have been formed, will set an end to the life of the plant and will rot and decay it. We shall do the same if we overboil and overcook our food. Instead of ripening, e.g. the leaf of the cabbage through boiling, we rot it when we expose it too long to the fire process. It is similar with the carrot. Here we notice that the carrot loses flavor and sweetness during the boiling, which tells us that Nature has fruitened the root in this case, that the "raw" carrot is not really "raw," but already sun-cooked; therefore we do often better to refrain from boiling it.

In other cases we may discover that the heat of the fire in the stove is not sufficient in itself, or that water is too inadequate a medium to bring about the ripening. If we want a quicker, shorter way to the fruiting stage, we can turn either to the fire-carrying tastes in spice and herb, or to the fire-bearing oils and fats. Frying and roasting, or stewing in fat, are then indicated instead of the boiling in water. Thus we have fire twice present, and if we add hot spices to the frying fat, it is even represented three times. Water is always a factor in all decaying processes, and if we want to avoid this during the cooking, we apply the concentrated, direct form of heat through roasting and frying.

Fire then is the great ripener, and in this capacity purifies and cleanses substance, but if this goes too far, fire becomes a destroying element killing life. This also is necessary in cooking, for on the way of being lifted up from darkness and heaviness to light and lightness, Fire has to free many bonds, much has to be dissolved, purified, even destroyed. Rampant life forces might overpower our digestion: as with the onion which when raw makes our eyes water, and braised in water will give flatulence, but when crisply fried, it becomes wholesome food.

On the other hand we should also not overdo the fire process and turn it into a mere burning of the food to cinder. As such it may be cleansed, but we have freed and sacrificed too much; what is left is mere ash, dead earth matter, and all other qualities have escaped and are gone for good. We see then that using fire alone, freeing alone, is not enough; we must also bind and fetter substances and qualities in our food.

As the Sun in Nature has the other elements at its side, so also the cook in the kitchen. The air, with its quick, evasive properties is the second assistant used by the cook for the fruiting and ripening of the plants. We meet it in conjunction with the fire of the stove and the fire of the fat in the roasting process. It is active in a still more direct form in all pastry work and baking. During the stirring of the dough we incorporate much of it, and we know well how particular we have to be with the stirring of the sponges, e.g., how their success depends on the fact that we have got sufficient air to keep the pastry light. Hot air from without and escaping air from within during the rising of the dough and the baking: this is the baking process. Yeast and baking powder as ingredients also do nothing else but give presence to the necessary air in a different way.

Other forms of supplying air are the many ways of stirring, beating, whipping and whisking. How the dish is lightened when we whip cream or the white of eggs! How different from the stodgy boiled potato are in appearance, consistency and volume of whisked mashed potatoes!

The air with its light weight, its thinness and expanding quality always escapes in abundance during all boiling, taking much of the food substance and aroma with it. In many cases this is good and welcome, and it is therefore often advisable (as with turnips or cabbages) to boil them with the lid open in order to give the air a chance to escape with unwanted substances and gases. Where, however, we want to preserve delicate flavor (as with fruit, broth, asparagus, cucumber), we do well to keep the dish well covered with a tight fitting lid. Here we want to keep the air prisoner, for we want to fetter substance.

The function of the water in cooking is as manifold and varied as in nature where it plays such an important part in all germinating, sprouting and growing, in the rising of the sap in the plants, in the falling of rain and dew. Water has no longer the expanding qualities of fire and air, but is already more akin to the earth upon which it falls following the contracting forces of gravity. Though water with its gentle coolness may be alien to the fire element which it also extinguishes when it has a chance, we cannot do without it during the cooking. Far from it: water is quite indispensable, for it must be ever present as the great combiner, mixer and unifer. Water has no form of its own, but moves and flows in perpetuity without having the escapist tendency of air. Water permeates everything. It softens and connects. On its waves so to speak all food substances flow together, meet and are united in one dish. Then they are carried by it through our own organism and are taken up by its own watery juices.

We see the water element appear during cooking when hard fats are dissolved during frying and in all other liquifying processes. We see it in the meat juices of the gravy. It is present in all fruit and vegetables. Their juices can be so abundant as in the case of spinach, rhubarb, tomato or marrow that they suffice for all boiling processes. Wherever Nature provides the watery element, the cook need not add any tap water for boiling or stewing. Water is also helpful as the gentle softener of all harshness, hardness and acidity: it mellows, tones down and dissolves. Where water as substance is not strong enough, the watery element in the form of milk will do wonders. Water as cook's assistant helps where fire gets too powerful, where this needs to be extinguished a little, be it the heat itself, or the sharp taste. It also assists in softening earthy hardness where air would be too quick, too light and would take away too much of the substance itself. Water is gentle in every respect, moderate, and we as cooks have often cause to turn to its mediating help.

The fourth and last element, Earth seems at first sight to be the one which has to be overcome and against which we have to fight in cooking, for so far we have mostly shown how to lighten solid, heavy, rigid form with the help of the other elements. That is, however, only one side of the true picture. When Nature provides us with hard, solid, harsh foodstuffs we have to free and soften them. But we must keep some 'earth' even in our softest, lightest dishes. We may have lifted it to a lighter, finer stage, but all food wants some solid matter, else it would dissappear entirely. However light a dish may be, something firm, something heavy and formed, something fettered by the gravity forces must remain. Little though this may be, the presence of some earthy matter must be achieved during the cooking. However watery or airy a dish may appear, it has 'earth' as a kind of skeleton within it. This we must consider in all our ways and methods of cooking. Our metabolic processes may want the weight of the 'earth' transformed, but the softening, cleansing and freeing must be arrested before the very end, the dissipation into the universe, is reached. What remains after that would be residue, ash, dead earthy matter which does no longer contain life forces for our nourishment. The elements must be on speaking terms in our food; one, the Earth, must not yet have fallen out with the others.

It can, however, also happen that there is not sufficient 'earth' in our food, then we try carefully to produce again hardness, firmness and form. It appears where we fry a hard brown crust, where we want crunchiness and a firm skin. Much of the frying and baking is done for the purpose of producing earthiness. We ourselves demand some hardness in an otherwise soft and sloppy meal, something to "put our teeth into." In baked puddings and cakes we produce almost an image of the earth herself, and it is most important to remember this when we choose the dishes for our menus.

Cooking, from this point of view, appears again as a great creative art and the task of the cook becomes an exalted one when we consider that she stands in front of the elements, the forces and plants of Nature like a great artist, choosing them deliberately, assigning to them their places and the parts she wishes them to play. Without the cook the four elements—so different, even antagonistic to each other—would produce an ugly medley and struggle of forces. She has to make them her friends and helpers, she has to balance them and to entice them to enact a play of beauty and harmony. Our meals in form and substance, in the deliberate choice of foodstuff and cooking process, will only then give us true nourishment and satisfaction when we thus learn to place them rightly into the great processes of Nature, when we see them as part of the sublime drama of human life between the forces of Heaven and Earth.

4. CONCLUDING REMARKS

Three great guiding principles have been the subject of the previous chapters, three pictures derived from plant and nature, which when considered and practiced will help us in all our cooking problems: the threefold nature of plant and man; the seven tastes; the four elements. It became apparent in each case that it is the cook's task to establish harmony between two polar tendencies in our life, between the heavenly pole of expansion and the earthly pole of contraction, just as in nature all living beings can only develop in a sound way when these two realms and forces are balanced and help together in unity. A trinity, a threefoldness, is established out of duality; a middle region is formed where the stream of forces from above downwards crosses those which are pushed upwards from below.

The creation of a threefoldness is the cook's aim, whether she selects the three parts of the plant—root, leaf, blossom—and gives them their due place on the menu; whether she aims at a balance of the seven different tastes; or whether she calls on the different elements for assistance during the cooking process. Yes, we could even say that always and everywhere in her dealings with food the cook has as her task the creation of a threefold plant. Once she may actually take the leaf part of one plant, a cabbage, e.g., the root of a carrot, or the fruit of the damson. But she may also create this new plant only by bringing into manifestation the forces of the three different spheres of which root, leaf, fruit are the most perfect representatives. Thus all that is mineral like sugar or salt, all that is hard and crusty, may be termed "root," just as all sweetness and fat, all softness and lightness may be considered of a flower or fruit nature. And what is of a mediating character and brings about a rhythmic exchange of contrasting qualities may thus be looked upon as a "leaf."

In this sense a clear soup can have the threefold plant within it as latent quality. The mineral of the salt and the bitter taste represent the root part, the salty flavor and the water the leaf, the fat and hot spice the flower. The selection of herbs for the bouquet garni for broths gives great scope for varying the nature of this new threefold plant. Even oatmeal is only harmoniously satisfying food if it has this invisible plant within it. The bitterness of the oats, the sweetness and cream of the milk, the salty flavor and watery consistency. A creator of ever new and ever varied ideal plants—that is the cook when she practices these three great guiding principles.

When now the work of the cook is finished and she has done all in her power to nourish and satisfy threefold man, her work can come to a crowning fulfilment only when those for whom the dishes were prepared, also eat them with understanding. It is one of the fundamental differences between man and animal, that he can eat while the animal feeds. The amount of nourishment we derive from food is enhanced, to an astonishing extent, by our attitude towards eating, towards the food and its ingredients. Man will develop his human qualities all the more if he eats with an attitude of loving interest and grateful reverence towards the substances and beings of nature of which he partakes. It is of less importance to man whether his palate likes or dislikes one or the other dish, whether he is partial to one or the other flavor. Let the cook trouble herself about that and let the eater trouble about the nature and character of the plants he eats. His loving and objective interest in the food substances, his understanding for their connection with him will contribute greatly to his being well fed and well satisfied. Man when eating connects himself with outer nature, he partakes of her forces and substances, of all that earth and heavens can bestow. It is an important—a nourishing and health-giving—factor of our meals if we think of this connection, if we meditate about it in an attitude of reverent gratitude before we partake of the meal. This is the blessing of the Grace, and Rudolf Steiner has given us one which in six short lines brings this great picture of Man in his relation to the World around:

The Plant seeds are quickened in the night of the Earth,
The green leaves are sprouting through the might of the Air,
And all fruits are ripened by power of the Sun.

So quickens the soul in the shrine of the Heart,
So blossoms spirit power in the Light of the world,
So ripens man's strength in the Glory of God.

(Translation by E. C. Merry)

5. RECIPES AND MENUS

A. RECIPES FOR THE AUTUMN

SPICY SOUP (For Cold, Damp Days)

1 tbsp. fat or oil
2 med. onions, chopped
½ cup leftover, cooked meat (roast or whatever is available)
1 bayleaf
paprika or cayenne
nutmeg or mace
basil
pepper   a pinch of each
ginger, ground
ground cloves
cinnamon
2 tbsp. flour
2 pints stock (beef, chicken or vegetable)
chopped parsley
chopped chives
1 tbsp. sour cream

1. Brown the onions and meat in the fat or oil. Add the spices and cook over low heat for five minutes. Add the flour and cook for another 2 minutes.

2. Add the stock and simmer for two minutes. Add the parsley and chives. Add the sour cream just before serving.

MARJORAM SOUP

2 tbsp. chopped marjoram
2/3 cup rolled oats or oatmeal
1 tbsp. fat or oil
2 pints stock (beef, chicken or vegetable)
salt and pepper to taste

1. Fry 1 tbsp. marjoram and the oats or oatmeal in the fat or oil until they are brown.

2. Add the stock, season with the salt and pepper and simmer gently until the oatmeal is cooked. Add the reserved tbsp. of marjoram before serving.

CUCUMBER SAUCE

1 cucumber
Salt
1 cup water
¼ tsp. chopped parsley
¼ tsp. chopped dill-leaves
¼ tsp. chopped chives
2 tbsp. flour
¼ cup water
salt and pepper to taste

1. Peel, clean and dice cucumber. Put in glass or pottery bowl, sprinkle with salt and cover with tight-fitting lid. Leave standing for one hour.

2. Melt the fat or oil in a saucepan and add the cucumber and the chopped herbs. Simmer gently until the cucumber is done. Add the water.

3. Mix the flour with the ¼ cup water in a cup and add slowly to the boiling sauce. Simmer for two minutes. Season to taste with salt & pepper.

Serve with meat, tomatoes or potatoes.

SAUCE FOR LEFTOVERS (OF MEAT)

1 slice bacon
2 tbsp. fat
3 or 4 onions, chopped
1 bayleaf
¼ tsp. peppercorns
¼ tsp. mustard seed
cayenne
cloves, ground
basil
thyme
sage, rubbed
marjoram   } pinch
lovage
chives
parsley
dill-leaves
fennel
caraway
¼ cup flour
2 ½ cups stock (beef or chicken)
salt & pepper & sugar to taste
1 tbsp. Worcestershire sauce
1 tsp. jam (damson, plum or other tart fruit)
1 tbsp. vinegar or lemon juice

1. Dice the bacon and fry in the fat for 3 minutes. Add the onions and fry until brown. Add the herbs and spices. Fry for a few minutes. Add the flour and fry the mixture dark brown.

2. Add the stock. Boil gently for a few minutes. Season with the salt, pepper, sugar and Worcestershire sauce. Add the jam and the vinegar and lemon juice.

3. Slice the meat and add it to the sauce, simmer until warmed through.

VEGETABLES

Beets

1. Clean, peel and quarter several large beets. Boil for ¾ of an hour in salted water. Drain and put through food mill or ricer.

2. Serve in a cheese, white herb, white onion or mustard sauce.

Yellow Turnips (Rootabagas)

Clean, peel and slice one large size turnip. Boil in salted water for one hour. Drain and dice. Serve in a sauce, such as one of the ones suggested for the beet, above.

Yellow Turnips

1 large yellow turnip
1 lb. sausage meat, or other chopped meat
    (for vegetarians, use herbed bread stuffing)
fat or oil for frying

1. Clean and peel the turnip. Parboil it whole for ¼ hour. Cut it, after draining, into slices ½ to ¾ inch thick. Cut out the center so that a ring, 1 inch wide remains.

2. Fill the center with the meat or stuffing. Fry the stuffed slices brown on both sides in a frying pan. Serve with gravy or a white sauce.

B. RECIPES FOR THE WINTER SEASON

CARAWAY SOUP

2 tbsp. caraway seeds
fat or oil for frying
2 tbsp. flour
2 pints stock (beef, chicken or vegetable)
Salt to taste
Pepper
Chopped parsley or chives

1. Fry the caraway seeds in the fat or oil until they are black. Add the flour and fry until this is brown. Add the stock and some salt.

2. Boil all together for five minutes. Strain the soup, add salt and pepper to taste and the chopped parsley or chives.

LEEK SOUP

3-4 medium size leeks
fat or oil for frying
¼ cup grated carrot
3 tbsp. flour
2 pints stock (beef, chicken or vegetable)
Salt, pepper & nutmeg to taste

1. Clean and slice leeks. Fry them lightly in the fat. Add the grated carrots. Add the flour and cook the mixture for 2 minutes.

2. Add the stock and add the salt. Bring to a boil. Leave to simmer until the leeks are done. Season with pepper and nutmeg to taste.

3. Chopped green leafy herbs may be added to taste.

LENTIL SOUP

2 cups dried lentils
fat for frying
1 med. onion, chopped
1 tsp. parsley
thyme
lovage
marjoram } a pinch of each
savory
basil
2 pints stock (beef, chicken or vegetable)
Salt & pepper to taste

1. Fry the lentils in the fat with the chopped onions and herbs.

2. Add the salt to taste and the stock. Bring to a boil and leave to simmer for one hour. Add salt & pepper to taste.

POTATO SOUP

1 large onion, chopped
1 tbsp. fat or oil
1 lb. uncooked potates, peeled and diced
1 carrot, diced
chopped green leafy herbs
2 pints stock (beef, chicken or vegetable)
chopped parsley
Salt to taste

1. Fry the onion in the fat until it is brown. Add the potatoes and carrot. Add some salt and the herbs. Cook for five minutes.

2. Add the stock and bring to a boil. Leave to simmer for ¾ of an hour. Season to taste and add the chopped parsley before serving.

HORSERADISH SAUCE I

1 large horseradish root
½ cup vinegar
1 cup cream
1 tsp. salt
1 tsp. sugar

1. Grate the horseradish root. Mix together the next four ingredients.

2. Add the horseradish to the mixture. Mix together.

Excellent with meat and fish.

HORSERADISH SAUCE II

3 tbsp. butter
3 tbsp. flour

1½ cups milk or chicken stock
1 large horseradish root
dried fruit (see list below)
Salt and sugar to taste

1. Make white sauce. Melt the butter, add the flour, cook for two minutes. Slowly add the liquid. Stir until it begins to thicken.

2. Clean and grate the horseradish root. Add to the white sauce along with the dried fruit. Simmer for 10 minutes. Season with salt and sugar to taste.

Dried Fruit: Currants, Grated apple (approx. ¼ cup)

RED CABBAGE

1 large red cabbage
3 tbsp. fat
½ tsp. salt
1 tsp. sugar
1 tbsp. vinegar
Water
Spices
Juniper berries (if available)
1 tsp. damson plum jam
2 apples (peeled, sliced but not cooked)

1. Remove the outer leaves and shred the cabbage. Put into a bowl and pour boiling water over it. Leave standing for 10 minutes, then drain. Fry the cabbage in the fat in a large pan. Add the salt and sugar. Cover and cook for half an hour, stirring from time to time as necessary.

2. Add the vinegar. Leave to simmer and only add as much water as necessary to prevent the cabbage from burning. Cook for two hours.

3. A half-hour before serving, season with spices, juniper berries and the jam. Put the apples in a layer over the top of the cabbage. Stir when the apples are done. Serve with any roast meat or fowl or with potatoes.

CELERY ROOT

Celery roots (Celeriac) may be washed and cleaned thoroughly. Boil them in salted water for half-an-hour and dice or slice them after draining. Serve them in sauce: White herb sauces made with parsley, chives or fennel; Cheese; tomato or light onion sauces are suitable.

KALE – One of the best winter vegetables which goes well with sausage, bacon, roast meat, with fried potatoes, or bread croutons.

KALE I

1 large bunch of Kale
1 onion
½ cup breadcrumbs
fat for frying
Salt & pepper to taste

1. Wash the kale and boil it with the onion gently in salted water for one hour. Remove the onion and drain it. Drain the kale. Chop the kale and onion.

2. Fry the breadcrumbs in the fat and add the kale, onion, salt and pepper. Cook for five more minutes.

KALE II

1 large bunch of kale
1 onion
1 cup oatmeal
Salt and pepper to taste

1. Wash the kale and boil it with the onion gently in salted water for one hour. Remove the onion and drain it. Drain the kale. Chop the kale and the onion.

2. Boil the kale and onion in a little water to which the oatmeal has been added. Simmer for half an hour.

C. SAMPLE MENUS

Boiled Beef
Horseradish sauce with currants
Potatoes
Brussels sprouts
Farina Pudding with jam *see recipe below

* * * * * * *

Potato Cakes
Beetroot with Cheese sauce
Spinach
Apples and Shortbread

* * * * * * *

Shepherds Pie (meat mixed with onions, herbs and grated carrots)
Greens
Pickled damsons
Stewed apples and caramel custard

* * * * * * *

Cold Beef
Potatoes
Beetroot salad with celery, nuts and spices
Apple chutney
Lettuce or greens
Blancmange (pudding) with Fruit sauce

* * * * * * *

Stuffed Squash
Tomato sauce
Lettuce or shredded cabbage
Potatoes
Fig or Date Turnover

Corned beef and macaroni with marigold petals sprinkled over the top
Brussels Sprouts
Grated carrots
Chutney or pickled pears
Plum Tart

* * * * * *

Cauliflower with cheese
Grated carrots with nuts and raisins
Lettuce or Shredded Cabbage
Potatoes
Chocolate Blancmange (pudding)

FARINA PUDDING

1½ cups milk
1 tbsp. butter
1/3 cup sugar
1/8 tsp. salt
3 tbsp. farina
1 tsp. grated lemon rind
3 eggs, separated
Jam

Put milk, butter, sugar and salt in saucepan. Heat to scalding. Add farina and cook, stirring constantly, for 5 minutes. Remove from heat and add lemon rind. Cool. Beat egg whites until stiff. Then beat egg yolks until thick and lemon-colored. Stir farina mixture into egg yolks. Fold in egg whites. Pour into 1-quart casserole. Bake in preheated moderate oven (350°F.) for 35 to 40 minutes, or until firm. Serve warm with jam.

III. FOOD FROM THE GARDEN

The Gift of Heaven
and Earth

by H. Hoogewerff

1. PREFACE

The aim of this little book is to arouse at the present time a wider interest in those edible and medicinal plants which are offered us in our everyday life. For what has been disclosed on this subject by orthodox natural science since the nineteenth century has generally arisen from a one-sided, rather material point of view, in which no place was reserved for the idea of forces as a spiritual activity, is sufficiently well-known. Matter was no longer recognized as a manifestation of spirit.

Our age is asking for a development of our knowledge from this point of view; for recognition of the importance (in addition to that of the quantitative material factors in our nutritive plants), of the function of those cosmic forces, which both heaven and earth bestow on the plant for its growth and development.

There may be some older persons who will consider it difficult to understand the language spoken here in connection with nature, but perhaps the younger generation out of their own individual thinking, will feel it easier to study the life of plants along new lines, especially where these concern the whole problem of nutrition.

Whatever our present-day ideas in chemistry about vegetable substances may be in their ultimate essence they are none other than cosmic forces, densified up to the state of matter, as these reveal themselves in the decomposing and composing processes of nature, where the regions of transmutation and demarcation lie between the airy, liquid and fixed elements.

In this short preface, the invisible mediators between *heaven* and *earth* which are represented by the chemical elements, have not been specially mentioned; it is, however, this activity which forms the background of this conception.

Neither can this be the place to bring forward anthroposophical ideas as to the differentiated action of the processes of life in nature of which I think I give here sufficient explanation in referring on the one hand to the cosmic (spiritual) activity of the life-giving forces of heaven—and on the other hand to the forces of the earth, which densify the life of nature into matter. With this conception it becomes possible to rediscover the presence of the forces from above, i.e., from the world of the stars and the energy of the sun working together with the earth in the power of the herbs to radiate light and heat, for man will find in the volatile oils of these plants forces which stimulate his own powers of life.

In the edible plants, however, the heavenly powers, in cooperation with the earth, so form the substance of vegetable food that man receives not only the "material," but the pure plant "forces" also.

Further one can learn to consider the sublimation of the plant substance, i.e., in the development of sweetness in flower and fruit, as dependent on super-earthly heavenly influences, as opposed to the quality of the earthly powers which bring about the mineralizing, cellulose-forming, densifying activity, as we find these in the hardened stem, in the wood of the branches, and in the root which holds the plant to the earth.

The indications given here are mainly in connection with the nutrition of human beings. They have been gathered together in the course of an intimate contact with vegetables and herbs.

2. VEGETABLE FOOD

The physiognomy of the vegetable kingdom is not really comprehensible until one is able to recognize it as a mirror of those forces of the heavens and the stars from which it receives, in cooperation with the earth, its infinite variety of growth, form, color and fragrance.

The plant can be regarded as a physical phenomenon, densified by the earth-forces, which in its form, though sometimes so transparent, fine and of so transient an existence that it would seem the earth with its minerals hardly existed for it; so slightly does it touch this earth as though only to give its roots an opportunity to attach themselves, whereas the plant itself rises up into the air, light and heat elements. On the other hand, we find plants that develop strong and broad forms with heavily enforced leaves growing robustly in relation to the elements and essence of the earth. This earth is often calciferous or it may in the course of time have become weather-hardened and of the nature of a greasy clay, or it may be loam or a fertile river silt. The plants in such soils receive nourishing elements, which enable them to acquire a luxurious, massive appearance. The leaves of these plants are rather hard and have often very strongly veined and ribbed leaves owing to the mineralizing forces of the earth, in the substance of the leaves. A typical example of this are the leaves of red and white cabbage.

When under the influence of heavenly forces the refined and transmuted vegetable-substances and juices densify themselves into calyx and flower, and a process of sweetening enters in, which manifesting itself in the formation of flower and fruit, and later in the case of certain seeds that develop sweet oils, the plant has purified the nature of its substance. What the *earth* gives to the plant is here being transmuted and sublimated by *heavenly* activities. The plant, as also the animal and the human being, must first destroy the nature of its food, in order to be able to build up its substantial form. What after all (generally speaking), expresses itself in the plant as it develops its flower and fruit, its scents and a variation of color, is the result of *predominating heavenly forces, and a partial withdrawal of the forces of the earth.*

The examination therefore of the plant's development from *germ-leaf via root to seed formation* will provide important material for the solution of our food problems. We notice for instance, how in all that is of the nature of *root-stalk and cellulose*, the forces of the *earth* predominate, whereas in the case of *flower, fruit, and seed formation*, the forces of *heaven* are dominant. In the leaf, nourished by the forces of air and light, we find the *principle of a preservation of balance* between the two.

From this point of view, we can understand that sugar from grapes, sweet fruits, and sugar-cane does not affect human beings in the same way as sugar from beets, the latter containing more of the hardening earthly element, though in the substantial composition there is almost no difference to be detected when chemically examined.

In the formation of seed, after flower and fruit have been developed, the earthly influences show themselves; the germinative power, the gift of heaven, densifies into matter and thus makes it earth-bound. The nature and the action of the grade of amylum is also different when we compare apples and pears for instance, with carrots. The vegetable world gives us more examples of this difference in plants, and parts of plants, which were either formed by the forces of the earth and thus bear its character, or under the influence of the forces of heaven have transmuted the vegetable-substance, thus presenting a product with a different "action."

By paying close attention to such differences one is able to a great extent to meet the needs of certain patients; it is also of great value where one is concerned with the food of infants.

What then we must ask is the proportion of heavenly and earthly influences in our nutritious plants in this scheme, *in which two poles which inter-penetrate each other appear?*

In the course of time every period of civilization has had its special influence, and many of our present day plants have lost their original form and character, so greatly has human culture changed them. As an example of what cultivation has made of the natural plant, we may, for example, study the various kinds of grasses, the Gramineae, which in their pure type are little visited by insects for lack of color and strong scent. One special type of Gramineae was chosen during the Persian era, by wisdom originating from the Mysteries, as suitable for making bread, and several species were cultivated.

Another example will be found in *chicory* (Cichorium intybus), in German the "Wegwarte," the one who "waits by the road side," of which Usteri in his "Pflanzensammlung" says, that in its wild state it only grows where human beings live. Partly chicory roots are cultivated as a substitute for coffee, or to flavor it. The remedial properities of this plant, at an earlier period, were also used in medical practice. It was only towards the end of the last century that the growth of this plant was developed by forcing into a long bud-like form now known as *chicory*, which is grown in the dark. The production of chlorophyl, which is dependent on the light-forces of the sun which give the leaf-vegetables their rich content of vitamins, have been quite shut off. This blanched chicory has hardly any nourishing value. Its nearest relative is our *endive* (Cichorium endivia) which originally came from Egypt. This plant when left to run to seed (by which means one can find the original form of all vegetable plants), can be recognized in its natural form, and with its big blue flowers will show a great similarity with the "Wegwarte."

Again, the *root-vegetables* and the beet family, of which there are many varieties, cultivated for their red, orange, yellow or white roots, are all types dependent on the human hand. Sometimes these root-vegetables are grown chiefly for their leaves, and then the roots have no longer the same importance, and the development of the leaves becomes of more importance.

In the sweet taste of certain beetroots (also in carrots), the bitter taste, which is characteristic of the salts of the earth, has been driven out and the sweet taste, caused by the heavenly forces, is found in the root, though the root, as such, remains earth-bound.

A slightly different process takes place in the *radish* (Raphanus sativus). Here also the cosmic light- and heat forces produce the root, which is accentuated in its rounder shape. The sharp and pithy taste is the result of certain freed sulphurous oils.

The horse-radish (Cochlearia armoracia), which originally came from China and Turkey, and in its wild state is also to be found along our coast, has a very different form, and its forces are much more vehement than those of the radish, which are rather like little subterranean flowers. In so far as it is grown for food, the growth and development of the horse-radish are also dependent on man's cultivation, which has cultivated it in such a way that its roots can broaden and extend themselves.

As a contrast to the generally cool character of root-vegetables, the horse-radish has a warming and strengthening power, because of the sulphurous oils present in the roots.

In the case of younger people, those of a phlegmatic, dreamy nature can be roused to inner activity by the use of horse-radish. But one should not over-estimate the help of herbal plants for human beings. With regard to the real values of different foods a spiritual insight—such as Rudolf Steiner possessed—was able to see their importance for human development. But nutritive values can never take the place of that activity which the human being has himself to carry out if he desires to take the development of his soul in hand for the balancing of his own nature.

The family of the *Brassica*, the edible *cabbage*-plant, (which originated in Western European coastal regions), form a transition from the root-vegetables to those vegetables whose growth is above the earth.

We will take the *turnip* first, which most probably came from Southern Europe, and belongs to the species Brassica rapa, a cultivated form related to the rape, usually grown only for seed, shows little similarity with the real character of cabbage and belongs rather to the tuberous-rooted plants.

Next in order we have the true *cabbage* species, the Brassica oleracea, which we find in numerous different varieties, now highly cultivated. Here the *Kohl-rabi*–(Brassica oleracea var. caulorapa), is a transition to the better known types of cabbage, which all of them show the remarkable earthly type, similar to the red or purple, green and white species of cabbage embedded in the upper part and resting on the earth, around which the stiffened leaves in the shape of a sphere closely fold over each other. The cabbage plants all have the typical character of plants which once grew by the sea; their hard, strongly-veined leaves seem to speak of the rough earth-water-element of the coasts and have nothing in common with the soft foliage of *spinach* which, nourished by light and air have a specially beneficial influence on the respiration and blood circulation of man.

It is well known how greatly the Brassica oleracea species were appreciated as food plants by the Greeks and Romans. The *"Wirsing"* or *Savoy cabbage* with its rugged leaves and more open "head" where the leaves are more loosely folded, also belongs to these.

In the case of *curled cabbage* or *winter-cabbage* the leaves have an altogether different form. Here the stalk is longer and thinner, and the free, loose, highly curled leaves form themselves into a kind of bouquet, (B. oleracea acephala).

The *Brussel Sprout,* in German "Rosenkohl," which put forth their buds above the earth like little roses, appearing regularly in the axils of the constantly rising stem, while at the budding points, the earthly forces have withdrawn more and more. The somewhat bitter cabbage taste is here ennobled and has become finer, more delicate and rather sweet.

One feels that the very different growth of Brassica oleracea, which appears in the *cauliflower* is somewhat unnatural, for here the Brassica has partly changed its motive of leaf-formation for the white compressed little bouquets, of its as yet unfolded flowers which have not anything in common with its mature blossoms that develop later. The taste of the cauliflower has still the character of a cabbage but has enhanced quality. The plant has, as it were, become oversensitive to the earthly influences, and is only able to develop in a well-fertilized soil.

The most interesting earthly appearance of the cabbage family is to be found in that well-known plant, the *rape*. This and the *earth-turnip* previously mentioned, belong to the same family of Brassica rapa, and represent the two poles of earth and heaven, between which the various typical species, which from root to flower have been gradually developed under the guidance of the human hand.

In the *rape,* we see the activity of the heavenly forces, which transmute its vegetable substances and show us their gifts in the fine quality and substance of the seed. In the high grade of volatile oils in this seed we can discover something of the earth-like nature of the plant. This is clearly recognizable in the honey which the bees gather from the flowering rape. It is the lightest in color of all honies, and crystallizes into a cloudly whitish substance. As it contains more of the earthly forces than many other kinds of honey it cannot by reason of its own nature, remain in a liquid state.

As a transition from the vegetables to garden-herbs we have to mention the *onion*, the Allium family, and Allium cepa, the *kitchen-onion* may be taken as a worthy representative. From earliest antiquity till today onions have been a cherished popular dish because of their purifying influence on the physical body. The *chive* (Allium schoenoprasum), so closely related to the onion, which is so much liked by the Belgian on his bread and by the French and Swiss people, for its delicate rush-like leaves. These are chopped very small and mixed with butter.

When the February mists pass away and one feels the coming Spring, this little plant rises from the earth, hardly noticed by the passer-by. It is a perennial plant, and will even grow on pure sand and spread readily. The aroma of its delicate light-power-giving leaves is not so strong as that of the leek (Allium porrum), which has the same forces, but much more intensely, and is more related to the earth. The ribbon-like leaves compressed to the extent of forming a stalk, and the hardened upper-parts of the leaves, which stand out like a fan-like shield, hardly give off anything of this aroma.

Indeed we come right down to the earthly in passing from the small hollow tube-like *chive*-leaves to the strongly-folded and stalk-forming leaves of the *leek*, somewhat similar to those of the *onion*. Whereas the onion rests in its spherical bulb upon the earth it is to a large extent penetrated by both cosmic forces and earthly substances. The *chive* needs a moist soil of sand and gravel, *leek* and *onion* prefer a limy soil. The *onion* completely unites itself with the earth. What takes place in the normal development of the onion, in its development of blossom and flower, and which can be compared to an inner process of combustion, through a metamorphosis and purification of the substance here takes place in the sphere-like form of the onion-bulb. Here the super-earthly-influences of heaven strongly penetrate the plant-substance bringing about a sweetening which is equally noticeable in the taste of the onion. When the onion is cut open and contact made with the oxygen of the air, it is the sulphurous oils of these plants (this also takes place in *chive* and *leek*, but not to the same extent) that makes our eyes water. In the thistle-like flower on the long stalk of the onion, we find a number of very small miniature onions which in autumn contain the black, oval-cornered seed, the *metamorphosis* of Allium cepa.

If we now pass on to the *shallot* (Allium ascalonicum), which came originally from Asia Minor, it appears as a variant of the well-known winter-and-summer-onions. Scent and taste are less strongly developed. Though now cultivated in Europe, this plant speaks to us of a milder climate and the influences of a different soil, which this plant has assimilated when in its original state. The *garlic* (Allium saturum), also came from the East. This plant is more sensitive to its surroundings, the taste is less pungent than our onion. Garlic is not so easy to cultivate as the other, as it does not easily tolerate the moist Western-European climate; its nature has more in common with that of the Southern and Eastern people, who use it every day.

3. THE LEGUMINOSEAE: PEAS AND BEANS

After the first-leaf vegetables, which the earth brings forth for our use from April and May onwards as food from the chill spring soil, it is only in the months of June, July and August that the *pod-plants* come to the fore-ground. The housewife knows all too well the work of shelling the first *peas* and stringing the *sugar peas*. The *broad-beans* too must be taken from their soft wooly beds and the *Kidney-beans* and the *French beans* freed from their strings.

The brown and white beans, the lentils, the green and white *flagolets* and the *butter beans* we eat in winter, ripen in the warm sun of July and August. In the seeds of these papilionaceous plants and starch and protein in which officially the nutritive values are to be found, are already present. If we observe their whole manner of growth, the rapidity with which they grow and develop, so impatiently and willfully do the tendrils of the peas and runner beans shoot up. This is really their original tendency; it is man who has influenced the more lowly growing kinds. In the quick germination, and in the irregular, quickly rising and twisting tendrils of the peas and beans, when we compare them with the more sober way of growing of the lentils, a definite difference of character in these plants appears. The stalks, which are usually flexible, seek supports to climb up and the spirals of the new tendrils often cling round the plant itself to grow ever higher. One might even describe the character of the peas and beans as eager and enthusiastic! Lentils excepted, have none of the inner dignity and restfulness of the *Gramineae*, the cereals which give us our bread.

By their strong relationship to the earth, the leaf-vegetables, the cabbage species and the root-plants must keep their growth more horizontal and have no power to raise themselves up, whereas the whole tendency of the *Leguminoseae* is to get away from the earth.

The *Lupins-species* and *Broad-beans* are exceptions, and give one an impression of a much closer relationship with the earth. The most important characteristics of these latter plants are to be found in their formation of flower, fruit and seed. The yellow lupin for instance would even prefer to produce its flowers and fruit twice a year, for before the seed has all fallen from the pods, the quick germinated young plant will appear and may even continue to grow till winter comes.

When, influenced by sun, moon and earth the new germ has gone through its preparatory stage, we gather the ripe pods and seeds and in eating these are nourished by their reproductive forces, by the starch and fats and the pre-eminent grade of protein of the *Leguminous* plants. The human organism thus reacts in quite a different way when making use of the peas and beans as when he eats the different leaf-vegetables and root-plants which are of phlegmatic nature. For this reason the popular mixture of carrots and peas taken together is right and beneficial. The more earthly nature of the carrot and the more cosmically influenced peas when taken together as food balance each other. Labiate-herbs, such as winter savory are especially valuable for preparation of the Leguminous vegetables because of these relationships.

This vegetable family of *Leguminoseae* asks but little from the soil in which it grows. By the sheer strength of its own nature even a poor dry sandy soil will satisfy it. The forces of light, and silicious elements provide it with sufficient food for the filfillment of its course from seed to seed.

The *Lentils* (Lens esculenta) which originate from Western Asia and the Mediterranean may be called the "phlegmatics" of the family for it is their nature to grow near the earth; and produce a humble pulse of a small brown roundish, and polished type. It is especially suitable for infants' food rather than the other pulses which have too strong an effect. Quite a different type of vegetable is represented by *Purslane* which is much used in cases of anaemia because of its iron elements.

Purslane—(Portulaca oleracea). When we see the purslane, with its thin stalks and pale green leaves, freshly gathered and arranged in a little basket on the greengrocer's cart, we do not see it in its natural form.

Originally a plant of the sea-shores, it still has the curiously irregular way of growth that we find in the wild plant today. We find it on heaths, in sand and sea-shores, spreading itself out in a dark crystalline shape; the four thick round red stalks which show the characteristic form of the plant, radiate from one central point and spread over the earth like a star.

Grown in a rich and fertile garden soil, and thickly sown, it grows richer in Holland on the heaths where each seed will tell to full advantage, the plant will sometimes attain a breadth of 50 cm. and more and will show its Portulacaceae-character, and a resemblance to the Mesembryanthemums will be discovered in the primitive structure of the plant and in the thickened, soft little leaves, which resemble those of the Sedums. The stalks are fragrant and have an acid pithy taste. When asked with what kind of herbs this vegetable should be prepared, the answer should be—*"with no herbs at all"*—it would be a great mistake, for vegetables like *Spinage Purslane* and *Endive* do not ask for any additional herbs when prepared. They stand, in so far as their taste is concerned, in between the "salt" and "acid" of the earth's influence and are in themselves complete in their high grade of nutritive value. Purslane loses much of its medicinal power and pleasant taste if treated as a green-house plant.

Here in the north we know it as an annual, the seed of which seldom ripens wholly and has to be imported from the warmer regions of the Mediterranean. Originally purslane is a stalk plant.

4. ROOT PLANTS

Who will fail to remember from their childhood the mournful evening cries along the silent streets and by the canals of *"Ramena-a-s* ramena-a-s!"* (Horse-radish). Then a poorly dressed peasant would appear with a bag on his back from which he would take and offer some black top-shaped turnips for a few pence. Later his *horse-radish* would prove when examined to be the inside of a very large radish, which is a treat when prepared in thin slices with a little pepper and salt, and is a favorite dish. In Autumn, it is the time of year for other root-plants.

There are young soft beetroots, both round or carrot-shaped, warmly red in color if not boiled too long, and served with some finely-sliced apples and with an egg sauce, or prepared quite simply with lemon, a little powdered thyme and some olive oil will make a delightful cold dish for supper. The thyme leaves, with their light-heat activity, balance the beetroot's strong earthly character, and as far as taste is concerned, will mix harmoniously with the beetroot. For a midday autumn dish one can take stuffed beetroots with nuts, and Coriander seed.

This season will also provide us with Celery. The young tender stalks are frequently served uncooked as *"hors d'oeuvres"* or with cheese at the end of a meal, and should be lightly skinned. It is usually served in a tall glass filled with water.

Another form of Celery is the bulbous kind called Celeriac which has a delicious flavor and odor, and is used either as a side dish or for making soup.

On the greengrocer's cart the first salsify now appears and the *Turnip*, also the more precious small white turnips, *"les navets"* which like to grow in a greasy clay, and are therefore largely grown in Belgium and Zeeland; they can also be well grown in a sandy soil.

The winter-carrot which can be eaten raw, but will also make tasty *"croquettes"* which are equally nourishing, and can easily take the place of veal-cutlets. *Wild mustard greens* can be taken from the soil the whole year round and kept in sand, not too dry.

The use of parsnip, a kind of white carrot, related to our yellow carrots but not so sweet, and with a more positive taste, has long been known as a very useful thing for making a vegetarian stew or soup, and is improved if a pinch of marjoram is added. The addition also of some raw grated carrot makes an excellent salad. Parsnips should not be cooked as long as carrots.

It has been said that a too frequent use of root-plants makes people stupid, but this is only the case if they are used in a one-sided way; moreover this applies more to potatoes, which are not roots but retarded stems.

If, however, we want to modify the earthly nature of potatoes we should prepare them with *herbs* and they can then be eaten without being harmful; for example we can add freshly chopped *parsley* or the warmth influences of the baked *onion* or grated charlock, coriander or caraway seed.

Kohlrabi—(Brassica oleracea, var. gongylodes). This delicious summer vegetable develops on a round-ish bulb just above the earth and thus provides us not only with its grey-green mauve or purplish Kohlrabi but also with green-blueish cabbage-like leaves, which can also be used, and can also be prepared like endives or chopped up. These leaves are sometimes rather tough and it is best to well stew with a pinch of chopped chives after the main cooking is done, or to give them a "Soffrito-treatment."

The Kohlrabi itself should be put on the fire, in cold, or rather in lukewarm water, and when sufficiently boiled, should be stewed for about ten minutes in a milk or marmite butter sauce with some thyme or marjoram, and then served. When the Kohlrabi bulb is very large, it can be cut into thin slices; a pinch of salt and pepper can be added.

Thyme, and also marjoram will then sustain the delicate aroma of the kohlrabi. The form of this plant is that of those stalk plants which are pressed downwards towards the earth, but without fully taking on the typical earth-character of a root-plant. When cultivated in hot-houses it will even quite lose its round shape and has a tendency to become more of a stalk plant in warm atmosphere. It then becomes woody. One can see with this plant, how quickly the shape of a cultivated plant, which is based on the balanced influences of the forces of heaven and earth, will lose either its original or its cultivated form, when one or other of those cosmic influences is made to predominate by an artificial treatment.

5. ON THE USE OF CERTAIN HERBS

"Man will once again learn how to use the herbs in
accordance with the development of his consciousness."

In order to study the herbs themselves more closely, especially that group which originally came from Central Asia, and was already known to the Egyptians and Hebrews, we can first take the *Labiatae* and the *Umbelliferae*. Though influenced and changed by a colder climate and other quite geological relationships such as growth on rocks, calcareous soil, or siliceous earth, they have been able to preserve their strong aroma throughout the centuries.

It may be said that the Labiates followed the stream of human history to the west and the north in the course of hundreds of years, and were to be found cultivated in many gardens in the middle-age. Today they are being grown again for their healing power, which together with other properties is developed mainly through a certain degree of radiation from the sources of light and heat. Apart from the fact that some Labiatae and Umbelliferae are chiefly used for medicinal purposes, the herbs here described are of value in the cooking and preparation of many dishes, and will much increase their nutritive values so that the food of human beings can receive their active influences in this way.

Only a few well known herbs are here mentioned. Considerable differences should however be noticed between such *spices* as which are imported from one or another of the different parts of the globe which are candied or dried, and the *herbs*, which have adapted themselves to soil and became native and less hot.

In the past the brotherhood of the Cistercians were great cultivators of *herbs* about which they had a deep knowledge. This order was also entirely vegetarian. In Holland as in the gardens of the monasteries of Egmond, Zundert, the Leeuwenhorts Abbey in Noordwijk and elsewhere, herbs were highly valued and were used for many purposes. At Zeeuwsch-Vlaanderen (a district near the Belgian frontier in the province of Zeeland) there was at one time a very important garden of herbs and oil-vendors and medical men from Hungary used to travel this district in search of herbs.

In Charlemagne's Capitulare de Villis the cultivation of these Labiates was ordered. Whether they traveled Westward from Central Asia over the Ural, Finland, the Scandinavian coasts, or went Southward along the South African coast, and the Canary Islands, or found their way along the Black Sea and Mediterranean to Spain and France, they kept always to the sea-coasts and their salty soil in which they could best flourish.

The unconscious relationships between man and the plant world in those days would naturally save him the key for their right application for daily use. Later the predominant intellectuality of human consciousness could no longer value the herbs properly, and the existing knowledge of their virtues. Chemical valuations of nutrition, chemically concocted medicines came to the front and the miraculous influence of these plants once called "Heavenly plants" (i.e. Salvia, Hyssop, Rosemary, Marjoram) by Nylant and Dodonaeus, retreated into a fairy world long ago known to mankind.

If we ask why the herbs have recently come to the front again today the answer may be that these things are connected with human development, with man's consciousness today in which a greatly increased interest in the use of herbs is now evident.

The whole movement towards reform in the sphere of nutrition has caused a reaction against the one-sided theories of the past century with regard to our food, though the old customs are still to be found surviving in schools and other institutions, where a certain quantum of proteins, carbohydrates, salts, and so on are considered essential even if a certain reduction in quantities may be noted when compared with some years ago.

It was the doctrine of those mysterious so-called vitamins which chiefly affected the development of the existing doctrines of nutrition as proclaimed by Liebig, Woehler and others. Though for so many people the secret of the vitamin has so far not been unveiled to the extent of any real recognition of the operation of cosmic forces, but still considering some beneficent substances to be bearers of vitamins, the human being whose consciousness is awakening and who strives towards further development where the daily returning food-problem is concerned, is now eager in his search for a different kind of food than what he used to get at home in his childhood. He is open to new ideas.

One finds also everywhere after the meat-eating habits of the past century, a leaning towards various forms of vegetarianism, the tendency towards raw food, the views of Dr. Bircher Benner and other food reform movements are accepted.

Among these different nutritional questions the herbs are patiently waiting for the time when they will again be rightly valued, both in the realm of medicine and in the preparation of food. The present day's rather negative attitude towards, and ignorance, of their usage has however not been able to diminish the beneficial operation of the herbs. Today they are needed for their nutrition, not so much for their material function as in earlier days, but for their gifts of light and heat-activity, which stimulate human powers of life.

The application of herbs in cooking must not be thoughtless and accidental; neither should it be from our pleasure in their taste and fragrance, for as in the case of other theories of nutrition, what is needed is a newly acquired and conscious knowledge of the function of the herbs we use.

If we contrast the plants well-known to us, in our common vegetables, cereals, fruits, and all that constitutes vegetarian diets with the place which the herbs and spices represent in the plant-world, we next notice in the previously mentioned vegetables, in their growth and development, a general tendency towards the development of substances. The vegetative substance-forming processes and forces predominate in these plants. We find them in the juicy roots, the fleshy stalks, the broad tender leaves, or the well-filled ears of corn.

Quite opposite chemical processes take place in the case of many herb-plants. One may even speak of an inner burning up of the vegetable substances through which a separating out of the volatile oils takes place which may be compared to a kind of secretion. When considered from the point of view of Goethe's doctrine of Metamorphosis in the case of some Labiates, i.e., Wild Mustard and other curative plants, one can say that in these herbs the etheric oils represent a prematurely completed process of development.

Further, when compared with the purely nutritious plants another tendency in shape and appearance can be observed. In some nutritious plants volatile oils also appear, but to a far less extent than with the herbs.

As far as the native herbs are concerned here in the north, the development of starch and protein is almost nil. In Asia and Africa, the cradle of many of our vegetables, the mutual relationship of food substances and volatile oils in one and the same plant may often vary, as it is dependent on soil and climate.

The effect of herbs on man varies according to whether they are added to the food when fresh or after drying; also if the food has been boiled or stewed. In the first case the herbs strongly affect the substances during their preparation, which generally improves dishes, and the human being benefits more indirectly. In the second case the herbs themselves act more directly on the human being and in their effects on the digestive processes. We know how the use of such condiments as piccalilly, mustard, English sauces, sambal (Javanese) produce a prickling burning sensation which may be good for tempting the appetite and stimulating the digestion. It seems as though the human being gets more easily through the process of digestion when these so-called "luxuries" are added than when he eats only rather tasteless and dull food, but their continuous use is not always good for healthy people for whom the use of these milder flavored herbs with their active powers of light and heat will equally well serve to stimulate digestion.

The different herbal aromas make the meal more appetizing and the hot condiments are no longer desired. For example we can take the
Dried Seeds of:—
Fennel (Foeniculum capillaceum)
Dill (Anethum graveolens)
Caraway (Carum carvi)
Coriander (Coriandrum sativum)
or the *Fresh Leaves* of
Chervil (Anthriscus cerefolium)
Parsley (Petroselinum sativum)
Fennel (Foeniculum capillaceum)
or either the *Fresh or Dried Leaves* of the Labiates:
Balm (Melissa officinalis)
Peppermint (Mentha piperita and Mentha viridis)
Basil (Ocimum basilicum)
Marjoram (Origanum Majorana)
Sage (Salvia officinalis)
Hyssop (Hyssopus officinalis)
Thyme (Thymus vulgaris)
Savory (Satureja hortensis)
Rosemary (Rosmarinus officinalis)
and other herbs.

When we make use of those parts of plants which contain the etheric oils, which give back the cosmic light-and-heat radiation they have taken up and *Transmuted in a Plant-Like Way*, these forces then unite with the food to which the herbs are added.

Moreover most of these herbs are able to preserve the existing forces of the food substances to which they are added during cooking or steaming.

Certain vegetable substances, however, are spoiled by long cooking or stewing for the natural forces which they contain have, when over-heated, a tendency to evaporate. Food should never be cooked too long. Here also the herbs can serve us well, for instance in the preparation of different kinds of flour, and such substances as are derived from plants cultivated with artificial fertilizer or have gone through some mechanical or chemical treatment by which their nutritive value has been lessened.

Dried peas, lentils and beans, which need a good soaking before they are cooked will be much improved by the addition of some of these labiate herbs.

Many of the root and stalk plants also need the cooperation of cosmic heat and light forces to tone down their mineralizing tendency before the human organism can benefit from them. This is especially so in the case of children, convalescents, or on occasions when the process of digestion should not be made too difficult. This does not mean that the use of herbs is always necessary. In many cases it is much better for young and healthy people to bite into a raw carrot than to eat them carefully prepared with herbs.

Neither do we need to use them with the fresh summer leaf vegetables, born of the cooperation of earth and sunlight so that all they can give us as life forces is already complete.

As a guide to the right use of herbs, the following diagram has been prepared.

The "Taste-spectrum", as indicated by Aristotle,[1]
elaborated and applied to the use of certain herbs.

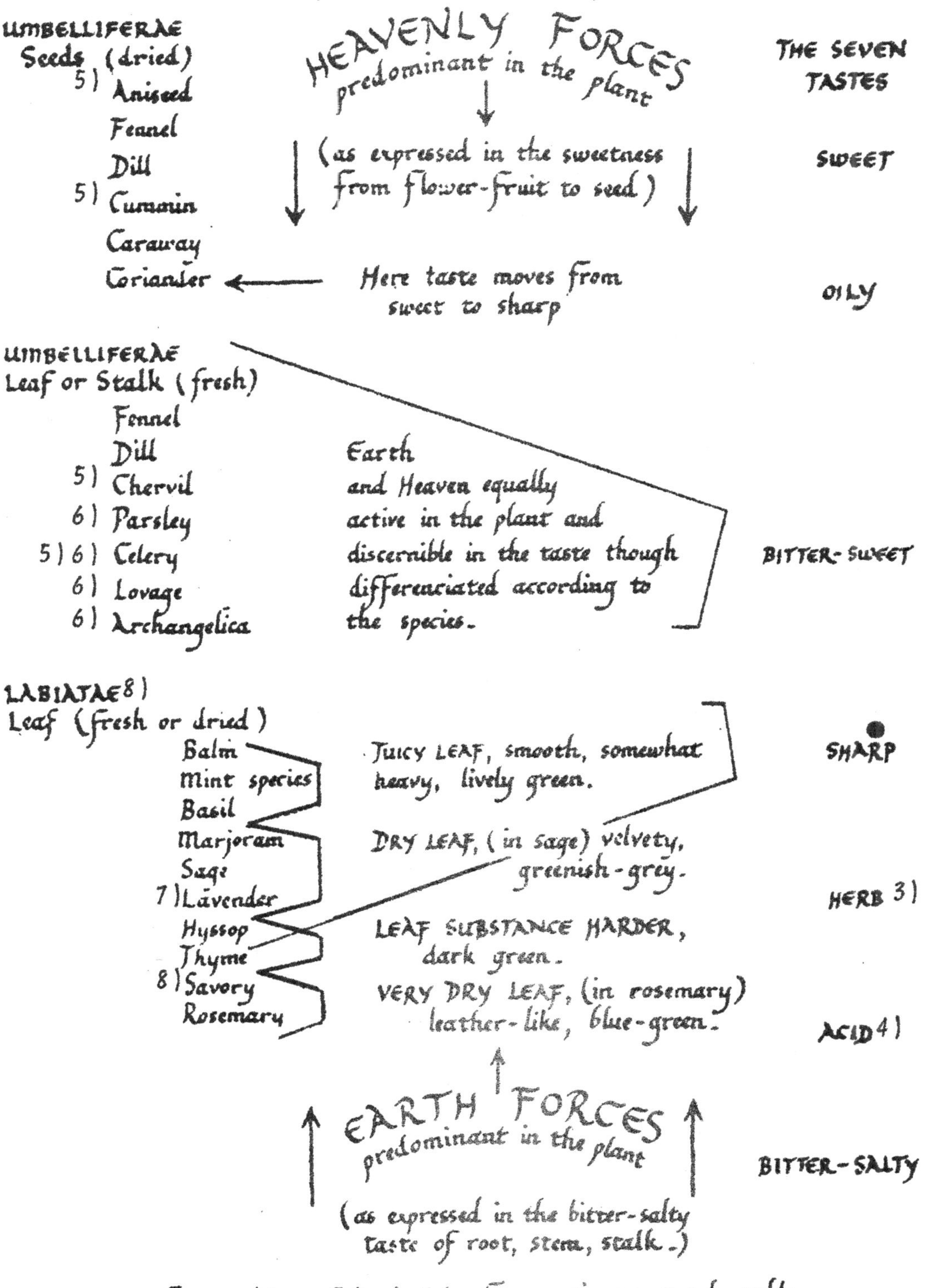

In speaking of "salt", in former times not only table
salt and what is by chemistry called salt was indicated, but
the densifying processes of the earth. Thus earth and salt had
one and the same meaning. In the taste-scale the bitter
salty taste is indicated in connection with the earth.

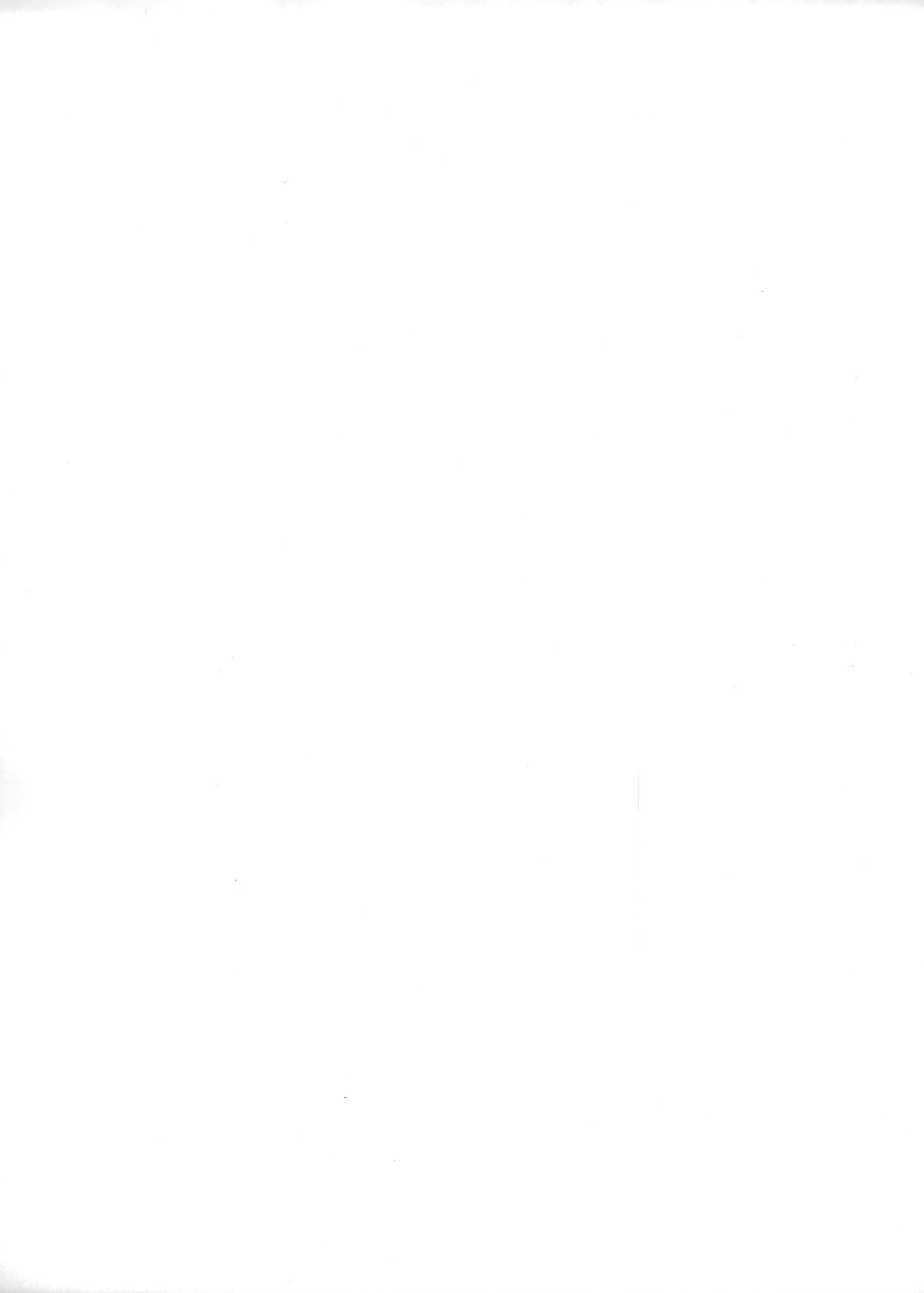

NOTES

1. Described by Ehrenfried Pfeiffer in "Natura," (no. 12, 1927) and here further elaborated.

2. Here "oily" is mentioned as the taste which may appear in some parts of the plant, when the heavenly forces predominate.
   a. As in the case of the etheric oils of seeds and nuts, when this appears in a complete state.
   b. Or in the case of etheric oils where the earthly substances are not completely sublimated, and the different aromas when considered from the point of view of the "salt" of the earth, show where the taste has not yet reached the stage of sweetness.

3. Here the German word "herb" implies something of a contracting nature. Herbs: les herbes (French).

4. The acid does not appear in any of the herbs mentioned here.

5. No recipes are given.

6. In the case of Parsley, Lovage and Archangelica the stalk can be used. If Lovage only a small piece of leaf for aromatizing the soup; of Archangelica only the young stalk should be candied.
   This series, once it is connected with any kind of food, should not be reheated, neither should such food be used the next day. Rather take fresh material again and again. (Archangelica is not taken in its fresh state for the preparation of food.)

7. Is not used for the preparing of food.

8. Labiates are less connected with the Earth than the Umbelliferae. One can notice this in construction and shape. They have a "herb" aroma. The seeds of the Labiates are without any smell, in contrast to the aromatic seeds of the Umbelliferae.

An answer to a question of how this variety of tastes can develop is to be found *in the way the plants and their organic parts are related to the salt and minerals of the earth.* There are herbal plants which develop more relation to the earth in themselves and are thus more dependent on this cosmic activity, and cannot therefore rise above bitter acrid and "dark" tastes such as we find in the leaves of Savory. The influence of the earth upon these plants is here stronger than the more purifying, liberating influences of the forces from beyond the earth.

When however, the taste is sharp and biting then both influences appear in a more regular way, as is the case with so many of our leaf-vegetables. The more the essential nature of the plant frees itself from the influences of the earth and allows the effects of the sun-forces to predominate in its processes of development, the more it will reproduce in its taste, the oily or sweet aroma we find, for example in roses and acacia and in many fruits. We find it also with certain nuts and seeds, but these again can become denser through forces of the earth. This is especially noticeable in the sweet taste of the Fennel seed though here also the volatile oils make their appearance, though originating at a different stage of the plant's development than the production of sweet oils. In the case of the Purslane, its harsh and acid taste bears witness that earthly influences predominate in this stalk-plant which also contains some iron.

In the "acid" of unripe fruit the earth is still active but is overcome by the light-activity of heavenly forces in the sweetness of the ripe fruit.

If we return to the plants, mentioned in the taste scale and picture their forms as they rise out of the earth searching for the air and sunlight, we come to Aniseed, Fennel, Dill, Cumin, Caraway, Coriander, the characteristics of which will be described later, and also Chervil, Parsley and Celery, the juicy leaves of which are not easily dried, for in these plants the more active are found in the juices of leaf and stalk and quickly volatilize in drying. When dried artificially these leaf-herbs lose their flavor after a few months, so that these herbs are mostly used in their fresh state.

They should not be cooked too long with the food and our best way to use them is to add them, freshly chopped at the last moment to the dish. The seeds of Parsley and Celery which have a strong taste, are mostly only used as flavorings and have no nutritive value. Archangelica belongs to this plant group. The stalk is well-known in a candied state on pastry of cakes. This plant, like Levisticum, of which the leaf and stalk can also be used in soup and is chiefly used for flavoring of Maggi products, but belongs rightly to the medicinal herbs. Both, when compared with Dill or Fennel, are of a much heavier and robust structure and more bound to the earth. The stalk is thicker, the leaves broader and stronger. The feather-like forms of Dill and Fennel can hardly be called leaves, they are so finely divided.

In the first group we have Aniseed, Dill, Cumin, Caraway or Coriander, which have a lighter structure and are less influenced by the earthly powers and more by heavenly powers. The seeds can be used in a dried state because of their cosmic heat-giving forces. Throughout their growth these umbelliferous plants seem to seek the flowering processes. Without their many heavenward directed umbels which develop on every stem with their countless number of minute blossoms, these plants would miss their most characteristic features.

The more primitive form of the Labiates is very different, for their typical characteristic is a more woody structure and somewhat thickset stature, the leaves are grey-green or bluish green, sometimes hairy, or rather dry, and for use in cooking or for remedial use the leaves should be gathered before florescence.

The lemon scented Balms and Mints have more juicy leaves. In the Labiates the leaves are less juicy and their rather woody stalks make them look rather like small Japanese trees, and the form of the flowers especially with those that have white or blue violet flowers give one the feeling that they are less typical than, for example, those of the Winter and Summer Savory, or of Thyme and Rosemary, which in their rigid structure give an image of the stiffening influence of earthly forces. In normal cases the influences of the heavenly forces reveal themselves in the development of blossoms, in the liberation of scents, but with the Labiates these essences are already developed in the small oval-shaped leaves which contain the volatile oils in their minute and invisible glands. When we arrive at the essential oils of this group of herbs, it becomes clear that the Labiates contain no poisons, a fact confirmed by the herbalist G. Hegi.

Whereas the production of volatile oils equally appears in other plants, this narrow and strongly aromatic leaf is typical of the Labiates. They can be dried quickly and easily, in really warm air in the dark. In some of these plants the aroma increases by drying; some of the labiate flowers are also fragrant, for example Lavender, Rosemary, Hyssop, Thyme, and here it is not so much the chemical composition of the volatile oils which make the Labiates so valuable for nutrition but rather the strong light and heat forces which the blossoms and leaves contain.

In cases where both a nutritive and a curative treatment is needed one may say:—

The human being, from the metabolic processes up to a spiritual consciousness, in many cases needs the strengthening and cleansing influences of herbs. They complete the food and even today though this is by no means appreciated by some departments of science, still bear the name of "Healing Herbs" and will assuredly confirm this title increasingly in the future.

6. FOOD PREPARATION

It becomes evident that in cases where an increased radiation of light than ordinary diet can provide, certain culinary herbs are necessary, a very modest amount of which will serve to increase the nutritive value of the food.

Each individual dish should represent a totality which should not only be rightly adjusted, but should also have a definite therapeutic value for the building up of the sick human organism. The selection of herbs suitable for each special kind of nutrition may be compared to the choice of the right colors and forms in the composition of a picture. Cooking and preparing food should be looked upon as a fine art.

The herbs should be added in very small, even in homeopathic quantities.

Their use for young and healthy children is not advised. When the child first asks for meat, the addition of a few soft herbs to the vegetarian food will generally divert any desire for meat.

It should be borne in mind that in cooking and stewing one is actually bringing about a kind of preliminary digestion of food.

In the case of turnip, potato, and some other root-and-stalk vegetables, and some of the more robust leaf-vegetables, cooking is an aid to digestion.

Such vegetables are often eaten sliced or grated, but it is not everyone who can benefit by a diet of raw food only, and in a damp chilly climate on an entirely raw-food diet, specially for young children or elderly people, should only be adopted on the advice of a doctor.

The whole secret of the right degree of cooking food is only to be found in a clear knowledge of the cosmic influences in relation to the balancing of the powers of the earth and of the heavens. It will be on these lines, which can be understood through a study of the plants themselves, that this whole question will be considered here.

In the case of ripe fruits, or tender leaves which are directly absorbed by the human organism without the assistance of any kind of cooking, we have the culminating point of what nature has received from the sun as a kind of "cooking." Further it cannot go.

Any further cooking or heating is only needed where there has been a deficiency of sun-forces so that a natural ripening could not be completed, either by reason of a lack of light and warmth, or from conditions related to climate and soil.

The *Root-Vegetables* do not need a sudden awakening from their earthly sleep to keep the cosmic forces bound to the root-parts of the plant, and should not be torn away from their natural state by too sudden and high degree of heat. They should be put on the fire in cold water. For young potatoes one should take boiling water or they will be reduced to pulp, for they have not yet matured to the stage of a fully developed stalk-root vegetable.

When a tea is to be made of *Blossom* and *Leaf-Herbs* like chamomile, mint, lime-blossom, and so on, a first drenching with boiling water and one minute's "drawing" is sufficient to bind the forces of the blossoms or leaves to the liquid and provide a fragrant "tea."

When cooking or steaming is prolonged the food loses its nutritive value. The life forces then leave the plants and little more than a dead vegetable substance remains. This has indeed kept its substantial characteristics, and these still have some value, but the supersensible cosmic forces, have withdrawn.

When preparing fruit (compote) also in the case of the finer leaf vegetables, a preliminary drenching in boiling water and a moment's boiling will prove sufficient.

Some fruits, also those of the *Leguminoseae*, which are often used in a dried state, need first the *Water-Element* and after that the *Fire-Element* for their preparation. Here the addition of water is more important than the heating.

Earth, sun-heat, and the influence of the planets are sufficient to provide for the pulses, peas and beans. In the latent state of their cosmic forces they need only the swelling action of the water to awaken and become active.

In the boiling down or preserving of roots such as ginger, stalks like angelica, leaves of flowers rose, or violet, petals, and many fruits, the normal grade of ripeness is overstepped.

They become mineralized.

With regard to *Baking* and *Frying* where a high degree of heat and fatty substances cooperate in preparing the food a rapid uniting of the food with its vital powers takes place which does not occur in other methods of cooking.

Apart from the fact that a light-brown crust forms over the food so that the nutritive value is preserved, oil and butter through their cosmic, heating activities will make the food more easily digestible.

It may be useful to give a description here of the so-called "soffrito" method. One cup of olive-oil, salad-oil or sunflower-oil should be brought to boil in an iron pan. Add half a chopped onion and the desired herbs and other ingredients. Chives or leeks can be used instead of onions, and parsley, celery or bay-leaves.

Here we have to do with a process of an intensive binding of these aromatic products which when complete must be taken up by the uncooked vegetables by a thorough stirring of all together.

If we take only some stalk vegetables or rice, a little liquid (vegetable broth or water) should be added while cooking. One often meets with these broths in Southern Europe, France and Belgium, while in Holland and England one finds a different custom, for in these countries the vegetables and rice are first boiled in water and the herbs are added later. An Englishman usually prefers to add hot sauces and pickles on his plate!

On the other hand a daily use of soup is typical for many continental people and especially in mountainous countries, where there is a desire for liquid food because these people live in a much drier and often warmer climate. People who live by the sea like the English and the Dutch, and have a more intimate relation to the element of water will therefore feel the need of a more substantial diet.

The French and the Belgians though their home is also near the sea, have none of the typical qualities of a sea people. So here we find the nourishing daily soup is prevalent.

Cooking in a *Double-Boiler*, a method in which the food does not come into direct contact with the fire, but is heated by water vapor, is actually an ideal treatment for custards, egg-dishes and such condiments, in which it is desirable to preserve the aroma of the herbs.

A still more intensive method is *Cooking By Steam*. This is especially desirable for stalk and leaf vegetables of a more earthly character. One can prevent many forces from getting lost by not allowing the vegetables to boil, but by treating them directly with steam-heat. Also when it is desirable to keep the vegetable-water for soups or sauces. There may however be cases in which one does not know what kind of fertilizers have been used in the cultivation of these vegetables, for when treatment with chemical fertilizers has been used the vegetable-water should not be kept; our whole mood and attitude when preparing food for others is also important and this even includes the way in which we stir or beat the ingredients—whether attentively or carelessly.

A rapid rhythmic stirring will help to liberate the forces and a beating up is necessary for all combination of lemon, egg and sugar. Lemon custards should be prepared in a double-boiler, so that the light forces of the lemon can affect the egg-substance, and lessen its more earthly forces in this kind of combination.

The *Preparation of Mayonnaise* on the contrary, needs a slow and regular movement of the hand which should cooperate with the earth-heavy sleeping element of the cold oil that here unites with the yolk of the egg and breaks it down. These oils, however, at the same time represent the highest development in the plant, and have been brought about by the forces of the heavens. Liberated by heating, the oil immediately loses its substantial heaviness, its *Forces of Light and Heat* awake and unite themselves with the food.

In such ways the human being, as he becomes conscious of the cosmic cooperation of the decomposing and composing elements in nature, and inherent in the forces of heaven and earth, the formation of which is dependent also on the elements of fire, air, water and earth, will be able to give intelligent guidance for the preparation of vegetable food.

It is evident that the kind of fuel used in cooking will also be important. Though it is unlikely that such a statement will be generally accepted by medical circles today, it can be said without hesitation, that cooking with wood, kerosene or coal, is much better than cooking with gas or electricity, though these may be easier for the housewife, who is not primarily interested in problems of nutrition.

The recipes which follow here, can also be composed with different herbs, such as tarragon, bay-leaf, nutmeg, curry and many others.

7. RECIPES USING HERBS

When preserving Sour-Kraut, Gherkins, Tomatoes, Cucumber and small Onions, herbs are a valuable addition, also when making jams from: Rose-hips, Tomatoes and other fruits.

Ordinary vinegar, which is often chemically made, can be improved by the addition of herbs, (bottom of page) or fresh lemon juice.

Puree of Tomatoes. The tomatoes should be cleaned, washed and sliced without adding water; then boiled with some finely chopped onion and one sliced lemon, well mixed together. Add a teaspoonful of dried powdered thyme and a little salt. No water should be added. Stir well and strain and the resulting rather thick puree should, before it is quite cool, be placed in a sterilized glass jar and covered.

Tomato Jam (sweet). This should be made like the tomato puree without water and boiled up for a few minutes only with half a sliced lemon, a teaspoonful of crushed coriander seed, sugar and a small piece of ginger. Put the mixture through a sieve and taste to see if more lemon or more ginger should be added.

Rose-Hips. When rose-hips are boiled down for Jam, a little dill seed, or fennel seed can be added to the sugar, also lemon juice and peel to taste. Put through a sieve.

White Onions. To pickle these take—1 part fresh peppermint leaves; 1 part basil leaves; ½ part pine needles; ½ part dried fennel leaves; ¼ part seed of coriander-seed; Add to the herbs 3 parts of vinegar, ¼ part of boiled water and a little sugar.

Gherkins. The same herbs can be used and a small piece of horse-radish added. The way to pickle these is to be found in cookery books. The gherkins should stay in the pickling brine for 8 to 10 hours before bottling.

Sour-Kraut. (In the proportion of two white cabbages or 1 green one.) Instead of pepper corns use a small handful of dried peppermint (stalk and leaf) and an equal amount of basil leaves between each layer of sour-kraut. Add some coriander seed. This will give the whole a fragrant aroma and help fermentation. Very little salt should be used.

Horse-radish and chives should always be used fresh.

Herb	Latin Name	Part used
Chamomile	Matricaria chamomilla	Flower
Fennel	Foeniculum cappillaceum	Seed
Dill	Anethum graveolens	
Caraway or Kummel	Carum carvi	
Coriander	Coriandrum sativum	
Citron-melissa	Melissa officinalis	
Peppermint	Mentha piperita,	
	Mentha viridis	
Basil	Ocimum basilicum	Leaf
Marjoram	Origanum majorana	
Sage	Salvia officinalis	
Hyssop	Hyssopus officinalis	
Thyme	Thymus vulgaris	
Savory	Satureja hortensis	
Rosemary	Rosemarinus officinalis	
Horse-Radish	Cochlearia armoracia	Root
Chive	Allium Schoenoprasum	Leaf

CHAMOMILE

Dried chamomile flowers make a valuable tea for bad colds and influenza. They can also be used for compresses. They are good for flavoring cakes and light pastries.

One of the herb gathering women, who worked here during the summer, wrote about this plant which has so slight a relation to the earth's forces. She said: "I feel the chamomile's flowers are real little sun beings. They have radiating little faces like tiny suns. They really seem to live with the sun. At sunset the flowers all close. At first I felt quite sorry to cut off all these little suns, but now I believe they like to give their powers of healing to man, for when one day we have almost gathered them all, the next day we find ever so many more radiant little faces welcoming us. I like to gather chamomile."

"Chamomile" Cake. 9 level spoons of butter; 24 spoons self-rising flour; 2 eggs; sugar to taste; chamomile—and caraway seed. The yolks should be well beaten with the sugar; add two tablespoons of chamomile-seed and one of caraway seed.

Mix well together, add the beaten up eggs and sugar and put in small tartlet tins. Bake in a moderate over for 20-30 minutes.

FENNEL

Fennel with its grass-green featherlike leaves, and dill with its somewhat similar, but blue-green foliage, have very differently formed seeds. The dill seeds are an oval shape and the best fennel seed has, like caraway, rather the shape of a crescent moon.

This plant, shows a balanced development between heaven and earth. One sees how the yellowish-white tap root which feels cold and moist to the touch, develops featherlike leaves which become finer and finer, more shining and more aromatic as the plant remodels the earthly substance, till, in the ray-like form of the flowers, it again transforms the seed out of the forces of light and air.

Fennel seed is specially good to use in preparing food for children, for example in porridge or in jam or when added to the batter for making thin pancakes. It has a sweet aromatic taste.

Fennel can also be used for flavoring sweet tomato soup. The fruits should be cooked first and passed through a strainer, then mix with butter and flour. Pepper and salt or sugar (cane sugar is best) can be added to taste. A few spoonfuls of grated celery, or celery seed are good additions.

Fennel seed is good to be added to a milky rice pudding, with or without raisins.

DILL

Dill-seed can be used to flavor macaroni, rice or any puree; also with white haricot or Lima beans or in the mixture for a cheese soufflé. It is also good with celery root, cut into slices, and the seed added when almost cooked. The slices should then be dipped into a thick paste made of flour and fried very lightly in salad or olive oil. Serve with a ring-shaped rice pudding. Add a sauce flavored with thyme or marjoram. Dill-seed can really be used to flavor any kind of pastry, and also with all steamed or boiled vegetables.

Apple Dish. Two teaspoonfuls of whole dill-seed and two of chopped dried basil leaves can be added to the butter in the frying pan. Then add one tablespoon of flour. Stir well together to a thick sauce by adding a little milk. Roll the slices of raw apple till well covered, and place them on a buttered fire-proof dish. Put in oven ten or fifteen minutes. This dish is good with leaf-vegetables.